Power Foods
for an
ANTI-INFLAMMATORY DIET

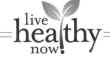

Beverly Lynn Bennett

live
hea|thy
now!

HEALTHY LIVING PUBLICATIONS
Summertown, Tennessee

Healthy Living Publications,
a division of BPC
PO Box 99
Summertown, TN 38483
888-260-8458
bookpubco.com

ISBN: 978-1-57067-388-7

Disclaimer
The information in this book is presented for educational purposes only. It isn't intended to be a substitute for the medical advice of a physician, dietitian, or other health-care professional.

Printed in the United States of America

25 24 23 22 21 20   1 2 3 4 5 6 7 8 9

Library of Congress Cataloging-in-Publication Data available upon request

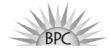

We chose to print this title on paper certified by the Forest Stewardship Council (FSC), a global, not-for-profit organization dedicated to the promotion of responsible forest management worldwide.

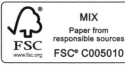

MIX
Paper from
responsible sources
FSC® C005010

CONTENTS

Chapter 1
Defining Inflammation

Inflammation is either the cause or consequence of nearly every injury, infection, and disease, and sometimes it's both. In a nutshell, inflammation is the immune system's defense mechanism in action. Under normal circumstances, inflammation occurs in response to an injury or infection and then stops once the problem has resolved. This is called acute, or useful, inflammation, and its symptoms are unmistakable. The root of the word "inflammation" derives from the Latin *inflammare*, which means "to catch fire" or "to burst into flames." This term encompasses the four symptoms that arise when the body experiences inflammation: redness, heat, swelling, and pain.

After an injury—whether it's a sprained wrist, a stubbed toe, a pinched finger, or an insect bite—all four symptoms will appear. Redness and heat indicate that blood is flowing to the location of the injury. Swelling occurs as plasma begins to fill the surrounding tissues. Pain is the telltale sign that something is amiss—a message the body is under attack and requires immediate attention. These symptoms are often acute at first but gradually dissipate as the healing process progresses. Eventually the body returns to normal, and in most cases, not even a scar remains.

Acute systemic infections (those that occur throughout the body) often take longer to manifest, but they elicit the same response from the immune system. With infection from a flu virus, for example, there might initially be a vague feeling of discomfort, followed by a burning in the eye sockets or joints, chills, and finally a fever. These are signs the body is fighting off the infection. Some people take anti-inflammatory drugs, such as ibuprofen, to relieve the discomfort. Others simply allow the fever to run its course and destroy the invading pathogen.

Allergies also trigger an inflammatory response. For instance, when people are exposed to environmental substances or foods they're allergic to, the immune system will launch an attack, causing symptoms such as a runny nose, itchy skin, or swollen joints. Usually these symptoms subside naturally once the offending allergen is removed. However, hypersensitive allergic reactions, known as anaphylaxis, can be life threatening and require immediate medical intervention.

Of course, more serious illnesses require more robust therapies. But in all cases, inflammation is the body's natural response to an invasive attack, and it usually abates once the healing is complete. Although the expression of acute inflammation can be unpleasant, it is evidence of a healthy immune system.

What Happens During Inflammation

When the body needs to respond to an injury, it mobilizes an army of specialized cells and chemicals to fight invading organisms and toxins. These specialized cells prepare pathways for fighter cells to attack and engulf the unwelcome invaders. Next, another group of cells signals the body that the fighter cells have been successful, which stops the production of the preparatory and fighter cells and triggers the appearance of clean-up and repair cells to clear the battlefield of debris and mend any damage.

Simply put, there are two stages to the inflammatory response: pro-inflammatory and anti-inflammatory. Each participating cell in the pro-inflammatory stage builds on the work of the previous cells and makes the immune reaction stronger. During the pro-inflammatory period, symptoms such as pain, itching, redness, heat, or swelling arise. The anti-inflammatory process puts out the fire, reversing the pro-inflammatory reaction and returning the body to normal.

A number of substances that either cause or block inflammation are made from essential fatty acids, which are fats the body cannot produce on its own. These fatty acids must be obtained from foods or supplements. There are two families of essential fats: omega-3s and omega-6s. Omega-6 fatty acids tend to increase inflammation; omega-3 fatty acids help to curtail it. It's important to remember that in a more complex depiction of the process of inflammation, some of these substances have multiple roles, including promoting the battle phase of inflammation and subsequently shutting it down when it's no longer necessary. The most common roles are explained in the descriptions that follow.

The Preparatory Substances

A number of different substances work together to alert the body there's been an injury. Other substances prepare the area around the injury to make it easier for healing substances to fight harmful invading microbes.

Histamine. White blood cells near the injury site release a substance called histamine, which increases the permeability of blood vessels around a wound. This signals fighter cells and other substances that regulate the immune response to come to the site of the injury. They gain easier access to the site because histamine makes the surrounding blood vessels more porous. Histamine also instigates swelling and redness around the site of the injury. Its effects are particularly noticeable during an allergic reaction, when symptoms might include a runny nose, itchy eyes, or a rash.

Eicosanoids. Eicosanoids are signaling molecules produced from essential fatty acids. They can be either pro-inflammatory or anti-inflammatory, depending on which family of essential fats they come from. Pro-inflammatory eicosanoids continue the work of histamines, increasing the permeability of blood vessels, which causes the swelling associated with inflammation. Prostaglandins are one of the primary pro-inflammatory eicosanoids; they make blood vessels more porous, create heat or fever to kill invading pathogens, and induce pain, which helps immobilize the injured area. Leukotrienes are another primary pro-inflammatory eicosanoid, and they also make blood vessels more porous and send signals to fighter cells to help them locate the injury. In addition, leukotrienes restrict airways and create nasal mucus, in much the same way that histamine does but more intensely. Pain is caused initially by the swelling that activates the immediate nerve endings adjacent to an injury. Pro-inflammatory eicosanoids increase the sensitivity of these nerves.

Cytokines. Cytokines are proteins activated by pro-inflammatory eicosanoids to signal fighter cells to gather at the injury site. In addition, they're responsible for diverting energy to the healing process. As a result, the release of cytokines may cause tiredness and decreased appetite because the digestive process requires a certain amount of energy and also supplies the body with energy. It's thought that the reason so many relatively healthy people died during the Spanish flu outbreak of 1918 was because that particular viral strain stimulated unusually strong immune reactions. Healthy individuals produced such high levels of cytokines in response to the virus that their bodies couldn't regulate the ensuing inflammation.

C-reactive protein. Cytokines, along with other pro-inflammatory eicosanoids, are involved in the activation of a substance called C-reactive protein (CRP). This is an organic compound produced by the liver that responds to messages sent out by white blood cells in response to infection. C-reactive proteins bind to the site of the injury and act like the surveillance team in a battle, identifying which substances are foreign to the body.

Many of the participating substances in the immune response are only present for a short time—just a few seconds in some cases. But C-reactive protein is an exception. Because it remains at measurable levels for up to two days, researchers and physicians often use it to gauge how much inflammation is present in the body.

The Active Fighters

Once the preparatory substances have readied a wound site, active fighters come into play. These microorganisms are responsible for destroying pathogens.

Leukocytes (neutrophils and macrophages). Several types of leukocytes, also known as white blood cells, are critical to the process of neutralizing invading substances. Neutrophils, which are small and agile, are the first to arrive at the scene of an injury to engulf and ingest microbes. However, neutrophils aren't able to digest all types of pathogens, so they're aided by macrophages, another type of leukocyte. Macrophages are larger than neutrophils and can tackle greater numbers of invading organisms. They have a longer life cycle than neutrophils, and certain macrophages also help with the repair process.

Free radicals. Both neutrophils and macrophages are coated with highly reactive substances called free radicals that kill invading pathogens. Free radicals are unstable molecules that trigger chemical reactions more readily than stable substances. Through a series of reactions, some of the free radicals on the surfaces of these leukocytes turn into hydrogen peroxide, and some of this hydrogen peroxide is then converted into hypochlorite—better known as chlorine bleach. Anyone who is familiar with these two substances will recognize them as lethal, not only to unwanted invaders but also to healthy cells. If there's any upset in the finely tuned balance of the immune system, which regulates inflammation and the production of these substances, there could be a resultant cascade of damage and disease.

Leukocytes are protected from the harmful chemicals that surround them because they contain large amounts of antioxidants, which are substances that neutralize free radicals. If the supply of antioxidants drops too low, leukocytes will become endangered and won't be able to fight off infection. However, if antioxidant stores become too high, the free radicals needed to fight infection will be compromised. In order for the immune system to function optimally and successfully, the many substances it relies on must maintain a delicate balance.

Reversing the Inflammation Process
Once the invading pathogens have been neutralized, inflammation subsides and the healing phase begins. According to medical researcher and biochemist Barry Sears, author of *The Anti-Inflammation Zone*, the overall inflammation process can be broken down into four stages: recall, resolution, regeneration, and repair.

Macrophages not only ingest invading organisms, but they also clean up the debris that remains after the battle, including any neutrophils that are no longer viable. The following are other substances that also play a role in resolving inflammation and repairing the injured area:

Cortisol. The adrenal glands produce cortisol, a steroid that turns off the activity of a number of the cells that prepare the body to fight infection.

Resolvins. Resolvins are part of a group of specialized compounds derived from eicosanoids, most of which are formed from omega-3 fatty acids, that tamp down the inflammatory response. Resolvins reduce the number of white blood cells circulating near the injured area and help encourage macrophages to clean up cell debris and toxins.

Protectins. Protectins are also formed from omega-3 fatty acids and are important for halting the production of prostaglandins and stopping cell degeneration. They are particularly active in the lungs and brain.

Chapter 2
What Is Chronic Inflammation?

Acute inflammation damages both good and bad cells alike, so the body keeps a tight check on it. However, for reasons not yet well understood, certain triggers can disrupt the fine balance that regulates the inflammatory process, resulting in chronic, or ongoing, inflammation. For example, when cortisol is released in just the right amount and for just the right length of time to stop the inflammatory process, this is a useful response. However, when cortisol is released, it circulates throughout the body, not just at the site of injury, and if it travels systemically on a regular basis, it ends up hindering the immune system overall. Not only will the continued presence of cortisol slow healing, but it will also heighten insulin resistance, leading to weight gain and negatively affecting brain cells that control memory. In general, chronic inflammation is particularly bad for the heart and brain because the cells of these organs are very slow to regenerate when damaged—if they regenerate at all.

Ailments Caused by Chronic Inflammation

Chronic, silent, or unproductive inflammation may be present in the body for years with no obvious symptoms. Think of it as a slow burn that goes unnoticed until considerable damage is done. Chronic inflammation follows the same process as acute inflammation, except it initially operates below the pain threshold and isn't temporary. If left unchecked, chronic inflammation can lead to serious health problems.

Cancer. Cancerous tumors secrete substances that attract cytokines (see page 7) and free radicals (see page 8), cells that cause inflammation, and use them to help the tumor survive. These substances also help loose tumor cells attach to new sites so they can grow and spread. When the body is already fighting inflammation from other causes, it can become fertile ground for cancer cell activity.

Diabetes. High insulin levels increase the activity of a substance called enzyme D5D, which increases production of the inflammatory omega-6 fat arachidonic acid. Consequently, inflammation can compromise the activity of the endothelial cells that line blood vessels, making it difficult for insulin to access other cells and help them take in glucose, which in turn causes insulin levels in the bloodstream to rise. Inflammation then creates a link between diabetes and heart disease: insulin activates D5D, which creates more inflammatory arachidonic acid and blood vessel damage.

Heart disease. Pro-inflammatory eicosanoids, such as arachidonic acid, can cause plaque inside an artery to rupture, attracting platelets that could form blood clots and aggregate to create a blockage. They also could cause an artery to spasm. Inadequate levels of omega-3 fatty acids can lead to an irregular heartbeat, which contributes to heart attacks.

Alzheimer's disease. The brain doesn't have any pain receptors, so we can't feel the effects that chronic inflammation has on it. Researchers have found that people with high levels of omega-6 fatty acids have a much greater incidence of Alzheimer's disease. In particular, the Framingham Heart Study showed that people with the lowest levels of circulating omega-3s had the highest rates of Alzheimer's disease, although researchers don't fully understand why. There is also speculation about the connection between Alzheimer's disease and diabetes; factors involved in insulin resistance also promote plaque development in the brain.

In some cases, the immune response will turn against the body itself. Autoimmune diseases, such as lupus, rheumatoid arthritis, and type 1 diabetes, are actually forms of chronic inflammation. Common symptoms of autoimmune diseases are allergies, asthma, chronic fatigue, joint pain, skin problems (including eczema, premature aging, and wrinkling), and even depression. Allergies are a form of immune response to various substances that most people's bodies would treat as harmless.

Chronic inflammation also contributes to and accelerates the aging process by prohibiting cell growth and regeneration. A 2014 study conducted at the University of Bologna that was published in *The Journals of Gerontology* showed how chronic, low-grade inflammation is inevitable during the process of aging. This relationship, called inflammaging, isn't yet well understood, but scientists do know that the greater the measurable inflammatory response in an elderly person, the greater the risk of illness and death. Gerontologists specializing in this area of research are exploring this association and are testing promising treatments that might help reduce inflammaging.

One possible cause of inflammaging is the amount of cell debris that accumulates as people get older. The body responds to cell debris as if it were a foreign substance, which in healthy individuals triggers macrophages that engulf and dispose of it. As we age, the disposal process becomes less effective, but the continued presence of debris causes the body to maintain an inflammatory response in an attempt to remove these unwelcome substances. Another potential cause is the action of the gut flora residing in the large intestine. During the aging process, the large intestine becomes more permeable and less able to keep these mostly beneficial organisms from moving out of the intestine and into the body; this migration may trigger inflammaging. It's also conceivable the organisms themselves might change in ways that cause inflammation.

Healthy cells are coded to prevent them from growing out of control, as happens with cancer. As cells age, this coding becomes persistent and prevents cell growth from occurring when it would be beneficial. Preventing unwanted cell growth is part of the inflammatory response, so cells that persistently shut down growth also trigger additional inflammation. Interestingly, cells that are signaling to slow growth are found in especially high levels in body fat, suggesting a link between obesity and inflammaging.

With age, blood coagulation capacity increases, which is also a part of the inflammatory response. This tendency may be responsible for the increased risk of dangerous blood clots in elderly individuals. The immune system may also experience the burden of a lifetime of toxic exposure, and parts of that system may decline while other parts become more active, contributing to inflammation. An immune system that is defective or functioning improperly could also lead to macular degeneration, one the principal drivers of blindness in older people.

People who live exceptionally long lives, especially those who do so in good health, offer an interesting counterpoint to the observation that chronic inflammation and aging are inevitably linked. The researchers involved with the University of Bologna study speculate that the usual methods for measuring inflammation might not be as accurate for predicting the potential for illness as was once thought. A small amount of chronic inflammation may always be present in the body, not as a response to illness or injury but as a normal part of cell death and regeneration. Also, some lucky individuals may have a genetic ability to create more of an anti-inflammatory response than other people do. As a result, they might experience less inflammaging in their later years.

The Causes of Chronic Inflammation

Chronic inflammation is most commonly caused by exposure to toxins and poor lifestyle choices. As noted previously, it can also be a natural component of the aging process.

Lifestyle Factors

Fortunately, many causes of chronic inflammation are linked to harmful habits that are within our control. By understanding how these factors influence inflammation, we can make positive lifestyle changes to improve our health.

More causes of inflammation are related to diet than any other factor. Top on the list of harmful substances are refined fats, refined carbohydrates, and animal products.

Although carbohydrates and fats don't contribute directly to inflammation, refined foods deliver a higher concentration of carbs and fats than is found naturally in foods. It's thought that these higher concentrations adversely affect gut flora in ways that increase inflammatory factors. When the body is in the throes of chronic inflammation, refined foods will have an even greater negative impact on gut flora.

The types of fats a person consumes can affect inflammation in a variety of ways. Before the advent of processed foods, the human diet had a nearly equal balance of omega-3 and omega-6 fats. Most modern diets contain much higher amounts of omega-6 fats as opposed to omega-3s, and in some cases, ten to twenty times as much. It's important to ensure an adequate supply of omega-3 fatty acids because omega-6s and omega-3s compete for the same COX enzymes, which are enzymes needed to build larger fat molecules. COX-2 enzymes in particular are essential for making inflammatory prostaglandins. If too many omega-6 fats are consumed, they'll dominate the use of these enzymes, decreasing the body's ability to build anti-inflammatory fats from omega-3s.

Fats that have been chemically modified can also contribute to inflammation. Early in the twentieth century, manufacturers sought inexpensive alternatives to solid fats. Because liquid oils were cheap and plentiful, food chemists explored ways to alter the composition of these oils to create solids. Their resulting discovery was what's now known as trans fats, which manufacturers used to make vegetable shortening and margarine. Unfortunately, no one realized at the time that the unnatural chemical structure of trans fats causes them to disrupt the normal flow of nutrients in and out of cell membranes and also allows harmful substances to enter cells. In addition, trans fats interfere with the action of COX-2 enzymes, resulting in the production of cytokines that signal the need for inflammation to begin, along with the release of C-reactive protein to assist the healing process.

Fats are also chemically modified when they're subjected to very high heat. When foods are fried, for example, toxic substances called advanced glycation end products (AGES) are created from both fats and proteins. After these foods are ingested, immune cells produce large amounts of cytokines in an attempt to protect the body from these harmful substances.

Animal products—especially meat and dairy products—contain higher amounts of pro-inflammatory essential fats, such as arachidonic acid, than whole plant foods. In addition, these animal-derived items introduce more pathogenic microbes into the body, triggering an immune response. Even when these foods are cooked at high temperatures or their pH is greatly acidified (such as by marinating them in lemon juice or vinegar), the toxins produced by the microbes they contain still exert an inflammatory load on the body. Also, red meat contains a type of simple sugar called N-glycolyl-neuraminic acid (Neu5Gc) that the human body is unable to process because it lacks the necessary enzyme. All other meat-eating animals carry this enzyme. Consumption of foods containing Neu5Ge creates an immune response in humans that is linked to certain cancers.

Other influential lifestyle factors include aging, hormone replacement therapy, obesity, lack of sleep, stress, and exposure to sun and toxins. As we age, fewer cells regenerate as they die, leaving behind more cell debris to trigger inflammation. Researchers at the University of Alabama found that oral estrogen can increase C-reactive protein (CRP) levels but that transdermal estrogen (estrogen that's applied to the skin) does not.

Adipose tissue, the layer of fat found beneath the skin, contains many white blood cells; the greater the amount of body fat, the greater the number of white blood cells present to release pro-inflammatory substances. Exercise releases myokines, which stop the action of pro-inflammatory substances.

When we don't get enough sleep, certain infection-fighting white blood cells, known as T cells, decrease, and the number of inflammation-promoting cytokines goes up. High levels of the hormones released during times of stress also trigger inflammation. Too much exposure to the sun (enough to cause sunburn) creates free radicals below the skin's surface.

Toxins that cause inflammation can range from dangerous substances in the environment to medications. Nonsteroidal anti-inflammatory drugs (NSAIDs), such as aspirin, ibuprofen, and naproxen, can stimulate or exacerbate leaky gut syndrome if used after periods of intense exercise. Cigarette smoke suppresses the capacity of white blood cells to produce substances needed for inflammatory healing.

Identifying Chronic Inflammation

Even if you appear to be in good health, you can suffer from "silent" chronic inflammation that hasn't yet manifested as discomfort or illness. That's why physicians often include tests that measure chronic inflammation as part of their routine physical exams. Most inflammatory mediators (substances that help regulate inflammation) deteriorate too quickly to be accurately measured except for C-reactive protein (CRP), fibrinogen (a soluble protein in blood plasma that helps form red blood cells), and white blood cells. The test for CRP and white blood cells involves collecting a blood sample; the results are often available in just one day. However, what's considered a "normal" level can vary from lab to lab.

Be sure to tell your health provider if you've recently been injured, had surgery, or undergone strenuous exercise. These factors can temporarily raise markers for inflammation and cause inaccurate test results, so it might be good to delay the test for a few days until your body recovers or normalizes.

Barry Sears, a pioneer in biotechnology specializing in the impact of diet on inflammation, is a proponent of testing the levels of two essential fatty acids in the blood: arachidonic acid (an omega-6 fat) and eicosapentaenoic acid, also known as EPA (an omega-3 fat). These two substances are the building blocks for the fatty acids that play a part in either promoting or reducing inflammation. Sears calls this comparison his "silent inflammation profile." Visit Nutrasource Diagnostics online at nutrasource.ca for information on where you can get your levels of these inflammation markers tested.

Chapter 3
How to Fight Chronic Inflammation

When most people feel the pain, swelling, and other common symptoms of chronic inflammation, their first impulse is to take medication, such as painkillers, antihistamines, or steroids, to combat their symptoms. Occasional use of anti-inflammatory drugs isn't associated with problems for the majority of people, but long-term use can cause side effects.

Nonsteroidal anti-inflammatory drugs (NSAIDs), such as ibuprofen and coxibs (Celebrex), work by interfering with COX-2 enzymes, which are needed to make prostaglandins, the inflammatory substances that cause pain and swelling. One of the most common side effects of these drugs is stomach bleeding. Less likely but still significant is the increased potential for heart attack, stroke, and liver and kidney problems. An alternative to using NSAIDs to treat inflammation with pain is to take acetaminophen, such as Tylenol. Acetaminophen carries less risk for side effects; however, it will only provide comfort and won't reduce the inflammation.

As the term suggests, antihistamines block the initial action of histamine, the first substance to participate in an inflammatory response. Antihistamines also block the activity of cytokines. Consequently, the drugs can be effective at the first signs of inflammation as well as hours later. Because H1-antihistamines interfere with the actions of histamine at H1-receptors, they are commonly used to treat allergic rhinitis, allergic conjunctivitis, urticaria, coughs, and colds.

Corticosteroids, also known simply as "steroids," such as cortisone and prednisone, are sometimes prescribed to reduce inflammation. These drugs are synthetic substances similar to cortisol, and, like cortisol, they can tamp down an inflammatory response. They are administered by injection, taken orally, or applied topically. In cases of dangerous inflammation, steroids can be lifesaving. However, regular use of steroids, especially when taken orally, is usually accompanied by side effects, some of which can be serious. In addition to stomach bleeding, which NSAIDs also can cause, steroids weaken bone and tissue, promote bruising, increase weight gain, and exacerbate mood swings. People with osteoarthritis and uncontrolled diabetes or high blood pressure should be particularly careful to avoid steroids or take them only under close medical supervision.

Natural Solutions to Curb Inflammation

Instead of blocking the inflammatory process with potentially harmful medications, use diet and lifestyle to reduce the causes of inflammation and increase the factors that inhibit it naturally. Dietary improvements will have the greatest effects overall.

The Right Balance of Omega-3 Oils

Anti-inflammatory drugs as well as fish oil (which is high in omega-3 fatty acids) have been proven to reduce cancer risk. Fish oil also has been shown to slow the spread of prostate cancer. It's safe to assume that a diet high in omega-3 fats would be similarly protective. Omega-3 fatty acids might help encourage apoptosis (cell death) only in tumor cells but not in healthy cells and make cancer cells more receptive to chemotherapy.

There's some evidence that anti-inflammatory medications taken on a regular basis can lower the risk of Alzheimer's disease. That's also true of a diet high in omega-3 fats, so adhering to an anti-inflammatory diet could be equally protective. For instance, older people who eat the most fish develop Alzheimer's less frequently than those who don't. Interestingly, omega-3 fatty acids have an easier time crossing the brain barrier than many drugs do; the omega-3 fat DHA is a building block for brain tissue. DHA has shown promise in improving cognition in Alzheimer's patients and reducing the development of brain lesions in mice.

The standard Western diet tends to be very high in grains, particularly wheat, which tilts the balance of fatty acids toward omega-6s. It also contains limited amounts of vegetables, legumes, seeds, and nuts, which are rich in omega-3s. Farmed food animals and fish are also fed an overabundance of grains, rather than the grasses or algae they used to eat.

To achieve a healthy balance, Western populations would need to move away from the processed foods so prevalent in today's modern diets and consume between two and four times as much omega-3 fatty acids as omega-6s. Research confirms that this ratio would still allow omega-3 fatty acids to access an adequate amount of the COX enzymes needed to make anti-inflammatory fats.

Many popular cooking oils, such as corn, safflower, and sunflower, are high in omega-6s. Better choices for cooking are extra-virgin olive oil and organic canola oil. Both still contain omega-6s but at much lower levels than most other oils. Although peanut oil and coconut oil are also very low in omega-6s, they contain no omega-3s. Oils that are high in omega-3s are flax, hemp, and walnut oils. Because omega-3 fats break down more easily in the presence of heat and light than omega-6s, store these oils in a cool, dark place or in the refrigerator and do not heat or cook with them. Oils high in omega-3s are best used in salad dressings and cold spreads or drizzled over raw or warm cooked foods.

Nuts and seeds and their butters are also good sources of both types of essential fatty acids. Those that are high in omega-6s include pecans, pine nuts, pumpkin seeds, sesame seeds, and sunflower seeds. Nuts and seeds high in omega-3s or that have a better ratio of omega-3s to omega-6s include almonds, cashews, chia seeds, flaxseeds, hazelnuts, hemp seeds, peanuts (which actually are legumes, not tree nuts), pistachios, and walnuts.

Those with the most omega-3s compared to omega-6s are chia seeds and flaxseeds. Walnuts contain more omega-3s per ounce than many other nuts, although they contain more omega-6s than chia seeds or flaxseeds. It's difficult to chew whole flaxseeds adequately enough to break them down, so if they aren't ground before they're consumed, the whole seeds tend to pass through the body undigested. Because any whole food that's broken down will expose the omega-3s they contain to damaging heat and light, it's best to grind flaxseeds right before using them. Alternatively, store freshly ground flaxseeds in an airtight container in the refrigerator for up to three days or in the freezer for up to two months; the ground seeds can be used straight from the freezer without thawing.

The Power of Phytochemicals

Phytochemicals are biologically active, non-nutritive substances in plants that help protect the plants from predatory insects and disease. Not only do phytochemicals protect plants, but they also impart similar protective benefits to people who eat plants on a regular basis. It's been theorized that organic produce may be higher in phytochemicals than conventionally grown food because organically grown plants need to develop greater natural resistance since they aren't treated with insecticides and fungicides.

When whole foods are refined, they're often stripped of the parts of the plant that contain the most phytochemicals. Cooking can have a detrimental effect on some phytochemicals, but heat can also make other phytochemicals more bioavailable.

Rich colors in fruits and vegetables indicate the presence of phytochemicals. The phytochemicals that have been shown to have the most potential for fighting inflammation are carotenoids (found in green, orange, and red vegetables and fruits), flavonoids (found in berries, citrus fruits, and soy products), polyphenols (found in berries, grapes, green tea, and whole grains), and terpenes (found in cherries, the peels of citrus fruits, and rosemary). Certain spices that are rich in phytochemicals, such as black pepper and turmeric, have been shown to help curb inflammation. The phytochemicals in red wine and red grape juice (resveratrol), blue fruits (anthocyanins), and turmeric (curcumin) can reduce levels of prostaglandins and cytokines. Although most phytochemicals are highly beneficial, a few, particularly alkaloids, might actually instigate inflammation in certain individuals. Alkaloids are present in vegetables in the nightshade family (eggplants, peppers, potatoes, and tomatoes), and some health advocates believe these foods exacerbate the painful symptoms of arthritis.

Avoid Trans Fats, Alcohol, and Caffeine

Don't consume foods that contain trans fats. These chemically altered fats inhibit the ability of COX enzymes to create anti-inflammatory prostaglandins. They also increase CRP (see page 7), especially in people who are overweight or obese.

Limit the use of alcohol and caffeine, both of which can reduce how much omega-3s can be used to create anti-inflammatory fats. However, because of the resveratrol in red wine, moderate amounts (up to two glasses per day for men or one glass per day for women) may offset any inflammatory activity promoted by alcohol.

Maintain a Healthy Weight

Inflammation has been shown to be higher in people who are overweight or obese. Body fat contains white blood cells, so an increase in weight increases the number of white blood cells releasing pro-inflammatory substances, which is directly correlated with a greater risk of diabetes. A diet based predominantly on a variety of whole plant foods, particularly fruits and vegetables, aids satiety, provides valuable fiber, and ensures a broad spectrum of inflammation fighters.

Limit Processed Foods

Avoid processed foods made with refined flours and instead eat intact whole grains. Replace sugar, sugary refined foods, and fruit juices with whole fresh fruits. A diet centered on foods that are naturally high in fiber reduces spikes in insulin levels more effectively than fiber supplements.

Consider adding naturally fermented foods to your diet. A growing body of evidence indicates that a healthy digestive system has a broad influence on overall wellness, beyond the organs of digestion. The intestines are home to a great many beneficial microorganisms, called probiotics, that convert nutrients and combat harmful microbial invaders. Naturally fermented sauerkraut and pickles are delicious sources of probiotics that help maintain a health-promoting digestive environment.

Include High-Protein Plant Foods

Many high-protein animal-derived foods—meat, poultry, and dairy products in particular—are sources of pro-inflammatory arachidonic acid. Although fatty fish can be a good source of omega-3 fatty acids, there are environmental concerns about our increasing reliance on fish as a protein source (see pages 22–23).

Most people are surprised to learn that nearly all vegetables and even fruits contain small amounts of protein, so eating a wide variety of them will add to overall protein intake. High-protein whole plant foods, such as legumes (beans, lentils, and peas), nuts and seeds (particularly walnuts and flaxseeds, both of which are also high in omega-3s), and high-protein grains (such as amaranth, barley, Kamut, and oats) can easily replace animal protein in the diet. In addition to the common beans most people are familiar with (such as chickpeas, kidney beans, and pinto beans), whole soy foods, including edamame and tempeh, are protein powerhouses.

There are many all-vegetable meat replacements in the marketplace, but these are best reserved for occasional treats rather than relied upon as dietary staples. The additional ingredients and amount of processing necessary to manufacture these products often makes them less than ideal.

Fish Oil: Not the Best Tool to Fight Inflammation

There's no question that fish oil, especially from oily cold-water fish, is an excellent source of the omega-3 fats that humans convert most easily into anti-inflammatory eicosanoids. However, the consumption of fish and their oil is problematic in several ways.

Common toxins in fish, including dioxin, mercury, PCBs, pesticides, and discarded pharmaceutical drugs, have become present in increasingly dangerous amounts in our oceans. Ingesting mercury at the levels often found in fish can cause neurological damage, while dioxin and PCBs have a host of adverse effects ranging from reduced fertility and immunity to heart problems. People who eat farmed fish instead of wild-caught fish in an attempt to avoid these contaminants might be surprised to learn that farmed fish often contain higher levels of dangerous chemicals than fish raised in ocean waters. That's because farmed fish are fed fish meal and oil from sea animals. Chemicals and toxins are stored in the fats of these animals and passed on to farmed fish in even higher concentrations than would occur in natural environments.

Even if these dangerous contaminants could be removed during processing, fish oil may not produce the results that claims suggest. Some studies show that large amounts of fish oil can increase the risk of colon cancer and may not have the protective effects against heart disease that was once believed. Other studies strongly dispute the claims that fish oil helps prevent Alzheimer's disease, cancer, and inflammation, or improves the immune system.

When weighing whether to consume fish oil, keep in mind the following two points: (1) Getting the right amount of essential fatty acids in order to reduce inflammation is a matter of balance, and taking high amounts of omega-3s is not necessarily a healthy practice. (2) The bounty of our oceans is at increased risk for depletion. The World Wildlife Fund estimates that the number of large ocean fish has decreased by about 80 percent over the last hundred years. Encouraging more people worldwide to consume increased amounts of fish and fish oil would ultimately make this situation even more dire. Because fish farms rely on supplies of ocean fish as a source of feed, eating only farmed fish wouldn't relieve this serious problem either.

The best alternative is to eat a diet that contains enough plant-based foods rich in omega-3 fatty acids to balance foods containing omega-6s. Freshly ground flaxseeds and chia seeds can be incorporated into cold cereals, salads, and smoothies. (Note that these seeds should be consumed shortly after grinding or stored for brief periods in the refrigerator or freezer to prevent degradation of their fragile oils.) Walnuts and dark leafy greens are also good sources of omega-3s. If you think you need additional omega-3 supplementation, consider getting it from the same source that ocean fish do: marine microalgae. Supplements made from microalgae are free of the toxins found in fish and untreated fish oils and supply omega-3 fats of the same quality.

Designing an Anti-Inflammatory Diet

A variety of anti-inflammatory diets have been devised by popular physicians and nutrition writers. Nutritionist Monica Reinagel developed a rating system that ranks the inflammatory potential of hundreds of foods. Her system takes into account the amount and balance of nutrients in a food, along with a number of other factors, including the following:

- the food's glycemic index (the potential of a food to raise blood glucose)

- the types of fat the food contains
- the amount of various antioxidants (such as vitamins C, E, and K, and certain B vitamins, as well as selenium and zinc) in the food
- how much of the amino acid homocysteine (a possible indicator of heart disease and Alzheimer's disease) the food contains

Use Reinagel's website (nutritiondata.self.com) to compare her rankings of various foods and determine which ones to emphasize in your diet and which ones to avoid.

The one drawback of using a ranking system is that it might encourage people to offset inflammation-inducing foods (such as meat and dairy products) with foods that have a low inflammation rating (such as cherries, chiles, and dark leafy greens). The best results will come from avoiding problem foods altogether and relying only on healthy ingredients.

Andrew Weil, MD, has drawn up numerous recommendations for an anti-inflammatory diet in his book *Healthy Aging*. Rather than zeroing in on particular foods, Weil encourages sufficient water intake and provides suggestions for calorie and fiber consumption as well as amounts and types of carbohydrates, fats, protein, and supplements (including particular phytochemicals, vitamins, and minerals).

Each plan has minor variances and presents somewhat conflicting recommendations. Evaluate them individually to determine which one will work best for you.

Chapter 4
Anti-Inflammatory Foods, Nutrients, and Supplements

You'll find some delicious, easy-to-prepare recipes in this book to help you maximize the benefits of inflammation-fighting foods. Nuts and seeds rich in omega-3 fatty acids provide the most protection, but a wide variety of vegetables and fruits also contribute supportive nutrients. The information that follows will highlight these foods and explain how they keep inflammation at bay.

Anti-Inflammatory Seeds, Nuts, and Oils

Many seeds and nuts are anti-inflammatory, either because they're particularly high in omega-3s or they contain substantial amounts of other nutrients shown to decrease inflammation.

Chia seeds and **flaxseeds** have some of the highest amounts of omega-3 fatty acids in the plant kingdom, with over 7 grams in one tablespoon of flaxseed oil and 5 grams in two tablespoons of chia seeds. **Hemp seed oil** contains almost 3 grams per tablespoon. **Walnuts** not only contain more than 2 grams per ounce but also contain phytonutrients, such as juglone and tellimagrandin (a tannin), that might fight cancers of the breast and prostate as well as inflammation in general.

Almonds were shown in a Spanish study to decrease C-reactive protein (CRP) and other markers of inflammation. **Cashews** are high in copper and magnesium, which can help control free radicals and prevent bone loss, especially in people with rheumatoid arthritis. **Coconut** (which could be thought of as either a fruit or a nut) contains medium-chain fatty acids that fight viruses and reduce inflammation. A Brazilian study found that the monounsaturated fatty acids in **macadamia oil** helped block inflammatory activity promoted by fatty tissue.

Be aware that certain nuts might cause inflammation, particularly in people who have an allergy or intolerance to tree nuts or peanuts. An intolerance may cause mild chronic inflammation but not be troublesome enough to arouse suspicion that nuts are the culprit. If you have digestive difficulties, try eliminating nuts from your diet to determine whether they could be the source of the problem.

Anti-Inflammatory Fruits

Berries

Blueberries, cherries, cranberries, raspberries, and strawberries contain phytochemicals called anthocyanins that have been shown to reduce several substances involved in the inflammatory response. Anthocyanins give these fruits their rich blue, purple, and red colors.

Research from Harvard University demonstrated that anthocyanins can lower heart attack risk by about one-third, particularly in women under fifty. According to research done at Oregon Health & Science University in 2012, tart cherries may have the highest anti-inflammatory potential of any food because of their anthocyanin content, and these levels may provide pain protection that's equal to some NSAIDs. Another study published in the *Journal of Nutrition* found that eating about one-half pound of sweet cherries per day reduced CRP levels.

Cranberries and strawberries contain significant amounts of polyphenols, another group of antioxidant phytochemicals that fight inflammation by reducing the buildup of platelets in blood vessels and lowering blood pressure. Strawberries also contain a natural anti-inflammatory called quercetin that protects against heart disease. In addition, the high amount of vitamin C in strawberries helps protect against asthma.

Açaí berries are small red berries native to South America and Brazil, and dried açaí berries have become popular worldwide for their nutritional content. A study conducted by Sloan Kettering Memorial Cancer Center found that açaí berries might suppress interleukins and COX enzymes.

Goji berries are bright red berries from Asia that have traditionally been used to promote longevity and vitality. Their active anti-inflammatory ingredient, beta-sitosterol, reduces the risk of heart disease, lowers cholesterol, and has a positive effect on enlarged prostates in men. See the box on page 28 for more information about goji berries.

Citrus Fruits

In addition to the vitamin C that's found in **lemons, limes, and oranges,** citrus fruits also contain limonoids. These phytochemicals slow the growth of breast cancer cells as well as colon, lung, and skin cancer cells.

Tropical Fruits

The leaves of the **guava** tree were the subject of a recent Korean study and were shown to reduce prostaglandins and COX-2 enzymes. Guava fruit is high in the antioxidants vitamin C and lycopene.

Succulent, green **kiwifruit** is high in vitamin C. It also contains a peptide called kissper that has demonstrated potential to reduce infections associated with colon disease, specifically Crohn's disease. Note that individuals with allergies to latex should eat kiwifruit with caution, as antibodies to latex can react to the protein in kiwifruit (as well as to the protein in avocados and bananas) the same as they do to latex.

Tropical **papaya** is rich in vitamins C and E. Papaya fruit has been shown to heal surface wounds, reduce oxidative damage, and increase the activity of antioxidant enzymes. Fresh **pineapple** contains bromelain, a mixture of protein-digesting enzymes that decreases cytokines and slows down the action of leukocytes to an injury site. It may prohibit the formation of cancer by dissolving the protective protein layer that surrounds tumor cells. Research done at Duke University found that both fresh and frozen pineapple were effective in decreasing the incidence and severity of inflammatory bowel disease. Bromelain has also been used to reduce inflammation from arthritis, sinusitis, sprains and strains, and surgery.

Other Fruits

A study done at Florida State University showed that eating an **apple** daily can decrease amounts of CRP by up to 30 percent. The fats in **avocados** help improve the absorption and effectiveness of carotenoids, substances that can inhibit the formation of inflammatory cytokines. **Rhubarb** has been shown to fight cytokines involved with systemic inflammation and may also be effective in healing cold sores and improving kidney function. (Note that eating too much rhubarb can cause diarrhea and stomach cramps. Also, rhubarb is not recommended in large amounts for anyone with a history of kidney stones.)

Nightshade Fruits and Vegetables: Arthritis Friends or Foes?

Nightshades are a group of plants that comprise a number of popular vegetables and fruits, such as **eggplants, goji berries, okra, peppers** (including **bell, cayenne, chile,** and **paprika**), **potatoes, tomatillos,** and **tomatoes.** Many of these foods contain high amounts of antioxidants, such as vitamin C and carotenoids (especially beta-carotene and lycopene). Chiles (hot peppers) are a source of capsaicin, a compound that is often used topically for pain relief.

Despite these benefits, many people believe that nightshade vegetables and fruits provoke inflammation (especially arthritis) instead of subduing it. Educated opinions about this are equally divided. The US Food and Drug Administration has stated that solanine, an alkaloid found in a number of nightshade foods, is poorly absorbed and therefore unlikely to be implicated as a cause of arthritis. However, a number of patients with arthritis have reported anecdotal evidence of a link between eating nightshades and an increase in the severity of their symptoms.

Since nightshade foods affect people differently, arthritis sufferers might want to eliminate them from their diets for a trial period of up to three months. After the elimination period, the foods can be reintroduced gradually, one at a time, to determine if any of them trigger or exacerbate symptoms.

Anti-Inflammatory Vegetables

Allium Vegetables

The allium family contains a number of pungent vegetables, such as **garlic**, **leeks**, **onions**, and **shallots**, that are known for reducing inflammation. Biochemists in South Africa determined that the sulfur-containing compounds in garlic may help stimulate the immune system to fight cancer, while Iranian researchers found that fresh onion juice reduced both acute and chronic pain related to inflammation.

Cruciferous Vegetables

Bok choy, Brussels sprouts, cabbage, cauliflower, chard, collard greens, kale, mustard greens, and **turnips** are part of the cruciferous family of vegetables. As a group, they're potent inflammation fighters. In general, they're high in vitamin C as well as other phytonutrients and antioxidants. A 2006 study from the Feinstein Institute for Medical Research showed that choline, a compound found in cauliflower, suppressed inflammation. A number of researchers, especially in Poland, have been studying the potential of sauerkraut (fermented cabbage) to fight the growth of cancer. **Turnip greens** are a good source of vitamin K, an inflammation regulator, and omega-3 fatty acids, the building blocks for inflammation fighters most often found in nuts and seeds.

Root Vegetables

Betanin, one of the most researched betalains, a class of antioxidant pigments, gives **beets** a high concentration of detoxifying substances that fight inflammation. **Beet greens** are also high in vitamins A, C, and K. The bright orange color of **carrots** comes from beta-carotene, which the body converts to vitamin A. Beta-carotene lowers inflammatory markers, particularly interleukin-6. **Rutabaga** is a good source of inulin, a substance that promotes the growth of beneficial digestive bacteria and a healthy immune system.

Jicama is a root vegetable popular in Mexican cuisine that is often prepared like potatoes. However, jicama contains fewer starches per serving than potatoes. As a result, it causes less of a spike in blood glucose levels and is less of a driver of inflammation. **Sweet potatoes** contain beta-carotene, fiber, manganese, and vitamins B_6 and C. Purple sweet potato extract has been shown to reduce inflammation. Sweet potatoes are an excellent alternative to white potatoes in most recipes.

Squash

The squash family encompasses a number of inflammation-fighting vegetables, including **summer squashes** (such as **zucchini**), **pumpkins**, **winter squashes**, and even **cucumbers**. In general, squashes are high in vitamin C, and orange squashes and pumpkins are high in beta-carotene. Cucumbers contain lignans that can reduce cancer risk and have been shown to block proteins that increase inflammation.

Other Vegetables

Celery is particularly rich in antioxidants, as it contains flavanols as well as the polyphenols caffeic acid and ferulic acid. **Celeriac (celery root)** is a source of vitamin C. Celery also is a good source of silicon, and both celery and celeriac contain vitamin K; these nutrients help maintain the health of joints and connective tissues.

Eating **mushrooms** is a gentle, noninvasive way to prevent metastatic cancer tumors and enhance the action of chemotherapy. White button mushrooms in particular have been shown to increase the formation of macrophages, the white blood cells that attack harmful invading microbes.

The protective power of olive trees can be found in **olive leaves**, **olives**, and **olive oil**, which is pressed from olives. Two phenolic compounds in olives, hydroxytyrosol and oleuropein, have been shown to help fight cardiovascular disease.

Consuming **soy foods** helps to reduce amounts of interleukin as well as tumor necrosis factor, a cytokine found during systemic inflammation. Whole soy foods, such as **edamame**, **tempeh**, and **tofu**, are more protective than highly processed soy foods. **Spinach** is a good source of the inflammation fighters carotenes and flavonoids. Spinach is also rich in the B vitamin folate and a number of minerals, including calcium, iron, magnesium, and potassium.

Other Foods and Beverages

Chocolate

Raw cacao powder is packed with antioxidants that slow inflammation, and these nutritious substances are more readily available in chocolate made with little or no added fat. Scientists now believe that beneficial bacteria in the large intestine convert the antioxidants in chocolate for use in fighting inflammation, but they caution that highly processed chocolate (even very dark chocolate) is not as effective as raw, unprocessed cacao.

Green Tea

The teas most people are familiar with (black and green) come from the same *Camellia sinensis* plant; the differences are due to how each type of tea is processed. Green tea contains more flavonoids, particularly catechins, than black tea, and therefore has a greater effect on inflammation.

Anti-Inflammatory Herbs and Spices

The concentrated oil from **basil** was shown in an Indian study to significantly reduce joint swelling in just one day. Researchers found that eugenol, the substance that gives basil its distinctive aroma, had benefits similar to several anti-inflammatory drugs but without the gastrointestinal side effects. **Oregano** contains carvacrol, an antioxidant that fights both inflammation and microbial infections, and rosmarinic acid, which helps protect against cancer. **Parsley** is a good source of myricetin, a phenol that blocks

COX-2 enzymes and cytokines, and apigenin, a flavone that helps to fight cancerous cells without harming surrounding tissue. **Peppermint** has antimicrobial properties.

The coriander plant can be used as an herb (**cilantro**) or a spice (**coriander seeds**). Both the fresh plant and seeds protect against inflammatory diseases that attack the nervous system, such as Alzheimer's and Parkinson's.

The spice that gives Indian food its distinctive yellow color is **turmeric**. It has a historic use in folk medicine as a pain reliever, and recent studies support the action of its active ingredient, curcumin, against COX-2 inhibitors. Piperine is the active ingredient in **black pepper** that provides its characteristic pungency. Researchers at Hamdard University in New Delhi found piperine to be extremely helpful in reducing the symptoms of rheumatoid arthritis. Piperine also helps the body assimilate certain medications and supplements and is recommended as a companion supplement to the curcumin in turmeric.

In studies of mice, extracts of **cardamom** reduced precancerous cells. The eucalyptol in cardamom was also shown to reduce gastrointestinal inflammation in rats. **Cinnamon** gets its flavor and aroma from a flavonoid called cinnamaldehyde. This substance will fight the growth of leukemia and melanoma cells and overall tumor growth. The anti-inflammatory effects of the active ingredients in **ginger**—namely gingerol and zingerone—have been widely studied. They've been shown to reduce prostaglandins, COX enzymes, and leukotrienes, particularly in relation to infection and cancer.

The Curative Power of Curry Powder

Curry powder, the distinctive ingredient in many Indian foods, can be a potent anti-inflammatory. The powder, which generally varies from household to household and cook to cook, is a mixture of many different inflammation-fighting spices, such as black pepper, coriander, cumin, ginger, mustard, and turmeric.

Using Anti-Inflammatory Foods

The best way to increase your consumption of anti-inflammatory foods is by using recipes that incorporate these foods as ingredients. In fact, it's easy to make dishes that include half a dozen or more different inflammation fighters at once. At the same time, it's a good idea to choose recipes that limit the use of foods that promote inflammation.

Plant-based dishes are strong in both regards. When fruits and vegetables are emphasized, dishes will automatically include many types of produce that contain inflammation-fighting compounds. In addition, using plant protein instead of meat, eggs, and dairy products essentially eliminates the inflammation-causing substances found in animal foods.

The recipes that follow are some of my favorites, and they're all inherently health promoting. To help you identify **the ingredients that fight inflammation,** I've highlighted those items in bold in the ingredient lists. Enjoy these recipes just as they're presented or use them as an inspiration for adding inflammation-fighting foods to your own favorite dishes.

Chapter 5
Anti-Inflammatory Recipes

Berry Blast-Off Smoothie

Makes 2 servings

Start your morning with a blast of energy from this smoothie. It's bursting with blue, purple, and/or red berries, along with other colorful fruits and veggies, which are all blended with omega-rich hemp and chia seeds.

1 cup water

1 cup fresh or frozen mixed **berries** (such as blueberries, raspberries, or strawberries)

2 large leaves red curly or Russian **kale**, stemmed

1 large **carrot**, sliced, or 1 small red **beet**, peeled and diced

½ cup **grape juice** or **pomegranate juice**

½ cup fresh or frozen pitted sweet or sour **cherries**

¼ cup **goji berries** or dried **cranberries**

2 tablespoons **hemp seeds**

2 teaspoons **chia seeds**

Put all the ingredients in a blender and process until smooth. Scrape down the blender jar and process for 15 seconds longer. Serve immediately.

Tip: If you're using only fresh fruit and would like a frozen smoothie, add ½ cup of ice cubes.

Indian-Style Tofu Scramble

Makes 4 servings

In this vegan version of scrambled eggs, curry powder adds both flavor and a yellow tint to crumbled tofu, which is cooked along with red onion, tomatoes, and spinach.

1 pound extra-firm **tofu**

2 tablespoons nutritional yeast flakes

1 tablespoon reduced-sodium tamari

1 teaspoon **curry powder**, or ½ teaspoon ground **turmeric**

½ cup diced red **onion**

1 tablespoon minced **garlic**

1 tablespoon **coconut oil** or other oil

1 cup diced **tomatoes**

3 cups baby **spinach**, lightly packed

¼ cup chopped fresh **cilantro**, lightly packed

Sea salt

Freshly ground **black pepper**

Crumble the tofu into a small bowl using your fingers. Add the nutritional yeast, tamari, and curry powder and stir until well combined.

Put the onion, garlic, and oil in a large cast-iron or nonstick skillet and cook over medium-high heat, stirring occasionally, for 2 minutes. Add the tofu mixture and tomatoes and cook, stirring occasionally, for 8 minutes.

Add the spinach and cilantro and cook, stirring occasionally, until the spinach has wilted and the other vegetables are tender, 1 to 2 minutes. Season with salt and pepper to taste. Serve hot.

Red Flannel Hash

Makes 4 servings

Savory hash is traditionally made from coarsely chopped leftover meat, potatoes, and other vegetables. When beets replace some of the potatoes, the dish is referred to as a red flannel hash, as in this plant-based version, which uses mushrooms instead of meat.

1 pound red **beets** with greens

2 cups (4 ounces) coarsely chopped button or crimini **mushrooms**

1 cup finely diced red or yellow **onion**

2 tablespoons **olive oil**

1½ tablespoons minced **garlic**

1½ teaspoons dried **basil**

1½ teaspoons **chili powder**

1½ teaspoons dried thyme

1 tablespoon nutritional yeast flakes

Sea salt

Freshly ground **black pepper**

Cut the greens from the beets and coarsely chop the stems and leaves. Peel the beets and cut them into ¼-inch dice.

Put the mushrooms, onion, and oil in a large cast-iron or nonstick skillet and cook over medium-high heat, stirring occasionally, for 7 minutes. Add the beets and cook, stirring occasionally, for 10 minutes.

Add the beet stems and leaves, garlic, basil, chili powder, and thyme and cook, stirring occasionally, until the vegetables are tender, 7 to 8 minutes. Add the nutritional yeast and stir until evenly distributed. Season with salt and pepper to taste. Serve hot.

Chipotle-Almond Mayo

Makes 1 cup

Whip up a batch of this egg-free, dairy-free mayonnaise, which is enhanced with a smoky chipotle chile. Use it as a spread for sandwiches or as a sauce or dip for raw or cooked vegetables.

½ cup plain **almond milk**

2 tablespoons **lemon juice** or cider vinegar

1 tablespoon **ketchup**

1 canned chipotle **chile** in adobo sauce, or 1 teaspoon chipotle **chile powder**

½ teaspoon **garlic powder**

¼ teaspoon **onion powder**

¼ teaspoon sea salt

¼ cup **olive oil** or **avocado oil**

Put the milk, lemon juice, ketchup, chile, garlic powder, onion powder, and salt in a blender and process for 1 minute. Scrape down the blender jar. With the blender running, slowly add the oil through the opening in the lid and process for 1 minute.

Transfer to an airtight container. Refrigerate for at least 30 minutes before using to allow the mayo to thicken slightly. Stored in an airtight container in the refrigerator, the mayo will keep for one week.

Bavarian Slaw

Makes 4 servings

The flavor of Brussels sprouts complements their cruciferous cousins in this slaw, which is coated with a Bavarian-style sweet-and-sour dressing.

2 tablespoons maple syrup

2 tablespoons cider vinegar

2 tablespoons whole-grain or stone-ground **mustard**

½ teaspoon caraway seeds

½ teaspoon celery seeds

½ teaspoon sea salt

¼ teaspoon freshly ground **black pepper**

8 ounces **Brussels sprouts**, shredded

2 cups shredded **red cabbage**, lightly packed

1½ cups shredded **savoy** or **green cabbage**, lightly packed

1 cup shredded **carrots**, lightly packed

⅓ cup thinly sliced **green onions**

¼ cup chopped fresh **parsley**, lightly packed

1½ tablespoons poppy or **chia seeds**

To make the dressing, put the maple syrup, vinegar, mustard, caraway seeds, celery seeds, salt, and pepper in a small bowl and whisk to combine.

To make the slaw, put the Brussels sprouts, red cabbage, savoy cabbage, carrots, green onions, and parsley in a large bowl and toss gently to combine. Pour the dressing over the vegetable mixture. Sprinkle the poppy seeds over the top and toss gently until evenly distributed. Let sit for 10 minutes before serving to allow the Brussels sprouts and cabbage to wilt slightly.

Tip: Use a food processor fitted with a thin slicing blade to quickly shred the Brussels sprouts. Note that shredded Brussels sprouts are sold in packages at many grocery stores; using them will make preparing this slaw even easier.

Berrylicious Spinach Salad with Raspberry Chia–Poppy Seed Dressing

Makes 4 servings

Chia seeds, rather than oil, are used to thicken this fat-free raspberry dressing. It's speckled with poppy seeds, then drizzled over a fresh spinach and berry salad.

1 cup fresh **raspberries**

½ small red **onion**, thinly sliced into half-moons

½ cup water

2 tablespoons cider vinegar

1 tablespoon **chia seeds**

1 tablespoon agave nectar

¼ teaspoon dry **mustard**

¼ teaspoon sea salt

1½ teaspoons poppy seeds

6 cups baby **spinach**, lightly packed

1 cup fresh **blackberries** or **blueberries**

1 cup fresh **strawberries**, cut in half and thinly sliced

½ cup alfalfa sprouts, lightly packed

⅓ cup sliced **almonds**

To make the dressing, put ¼ cup of the raspberries, 1 tablespoon of the onion, and the water, vinegar, chia seeds, agave nectar, dry mustard, and salt in a blender and process for 1 minute. Transfer the dressing to a small bowl and stir in the poppy seeds.

To make the salad, put the spinach, remaining raspberries and onion, and the blackberries and strawberries in a large bowl and toss to combine. Scatter the sprouts and almonds over the top. Drizzle the dressing over each serving.

Mexicali Veggie Chili

Makes 6 servings

This thick and hearty chili is packed with a colorful assortment of diced vegetables, crushed tomatoes, two kinds of beans, and cacao powder, which, surprisingly, deepens the flavor of the chili.

1 red or yellow **onion**, diced

1 red, orange, or yellow **bell pepper**, diced

1 **sweet potato**, peeled and diced

1 small **zucchini**, diced

1 small **yellow squash**, diced

1½ tablespoons **olive oil**

1 jalapeño **chile**, seeded and finely diced (optional)

2 tablespoons minced **garlic**

1½ teaspoons **chili powder**

1½ teaspoons dried **oregano**

1 teaspoon ground **cumin**

¼ teaspoon **cayenne** or chipotle **chile powder** (optional)

1 can (28 ounces) crushed **tomatoes**

1 can (15 ounces) black beans, drained and rinsed

1 can (15 ounces) kidney beans, drained and rinsed

1½ cups water

1 tablespoon **unsweetened cocoa powder**

⅓ cup chopped fresh **cilantro**, lightly packed

Sea salt

Freshly ground **black pepper**

1 **avocado**, diced

Hot sauce (optional)

Put the onion, bell pepper, sweet potato, zucchini, yellow squash, and oil in a large soup pot and cook, stirring occasionally, for 10 minutes. Add the chile, garlic, chili powder, oregano, cumin, and optional cayenne and cook, stirring occasionally, for 2 minutes.

Add the tomatoes, black beans, kidney beans, water, and cacao powder and stir to combine. Bring to a boil over high heat. Cover, decrease the heat to low, and simmer, stirring occasionally, until the vegetables are tender, about 30 minutes. Add the cilantro and stir until evenly distributed. Season with salt and pepper to taste. Garnish each serving with some of the avocado and a little hot sauce if desired. Serve hot.

Creole-Style Sweet Potato Skillet

Makes 4 servings

In the Creole cuisine of Louisiana, the combination of bell pepper, onion, and celery is often referred to as the "holy trinity." This flavor-enhancing blend unites with sweet potatoes, collard greens, and green onions in this mix, along with some jalapeño chiles and cayenne for a little heat to round out the flavors.

1 cup diced red or yellow **bell pepper**

1 cup diced yellow **onion**

2 stalks **celery**, diced

2 tablespoons **olive oil**

2½ cups peeled and finely diced **sweet potatoes**

½ cup thinly sliced **green onions**

2 jalapeño **chiles**, cut in half lengthwise, seeded, and thinly sliced

1 tablespoon minced **garlic**

1½ teaspoons dried thyme

½ teaspoon **cayenne**

2 cups stemmed and thinly sliced **collard greens**, lightly packed

Sea salt

Freshly ground **black pepper**

Put the bell pepper, onion, celery, and oil in a large cast-iron or nonstick skillet and cook over medium-high heat, stirring occasionally, for 5 minutes. Add the sweet potatoes and cook, stirring occasionally, for 8 minutes.

Add the green onions, chiles, garlic, thyme, and cayenne and cook, stirring occasionally, for 2 minutes. Add the collard greens and cook, stirring occasionally, until the greens have wilted and the other vegetables are tender, 3 to 5 minutes. Season with salt and pepper to taste. Serve hot.

Squash and Cherry Tomato Medley with Olives

Makes 4 servings

The flavors and textures of summer squash, zucchini, and cherry tomatoes complement each other beautifully. This colorful combination is further enhanced with the addition of salty olives and fresh herbs.

2 **yellow squashes**, cut in half lengthwise and sliced into ½-inch-thick half-moons

2 **zucchini**, cut in half lengthwise and sliced into ½-inch-thick half-moons

1 tablespoon **olive oil**

3 cups cherry **tomatoes**

½ cup pitted green or black **olives** or a combination, cut in half

2 tablespoons minced **garlic**

⅓ cup chopped fresh **basil**, lightly packed

2 tablespoons chopped fresh marjoram or **oregano**, or 2 teaspoons dried

1½ tablespoons nutritional yeast flakes

Sea salt

Freshly ground **black pepper**

Put the yellow squashes, zucchini, and oil in a large cast-iron or nonstick skillet and cook over medium-high heat, stirring occasionally, for 5 minutes. Add the tomatoes, olives, and garlic and cook, stirring occasionally, until the yellow squashes and zucchini are crisp-tender and the tomatoes are just starting to soften and release their juices, about 3 minutes.

Add the basil, marjoram, and nutritional yeast and stir until evenly distributed. Season with salt and pepper to taste. Serve hot.

Maple-Glazed Winter Squash

Makes 6 servings

Winter squashes abound during the colder months of the year. To make the most of this bounty, give this simple, quick recipe a try. It features tender cubes of winter squash covered in a spiced glaze made with maple syrup and coconut oil.

> 1 large (about 3 pounds) **winter squash**, peeled, seeded, and cut into 1-inch cubes
> 1½ cups water
> 1½ tablespoons peeled and grated fresh **ginger**
> 3 tablespoons maple syrup
> 1 tablespoon **coconut oil**, melted
> 1 teaspoon ground **cinnamon**
> Sea salt

Put the squash, water, and ginger in a large cast-iron or nonstick skillet. Cover and cook over medium heat until the squash is tender, 15 to 20 minutes. Remove the lid. Add the maple syrup, oil, and cinnamon and cook, stirring occasionally, until the cooking liquid thickens to a glaze. Remove from the heat. Season with salt to taste. Serve hot.

CHAPTER 5: ANTI-INFLAMMATORY RECIPES **45**

Spicy Sweet Potato Fries

Makes 4 servings

Oven-baked fries use just a fraction of the fat as their deep-fried counterparts, which means you can still get your French-fry fix but with less guilt. For a first-rate batch of oven-baked fries, coat sweet potato strips generously with a blend of spices, then bake them until crisp and tender. Chipotle-Almond Mayo (page 37) is an excellent dipping sauce for these spicy fries.

5 cups (2 large) **sweet potatoes**, scrubbed well and cut into
    3 x ½-inch French fries

1½ tablespoons **olive oil**

1½ tablespoons nutritional yeast flakes

2 teaspoons **chili powder**

1 teaspoon ground **cumin**

1 teaspoon **garlic powder**

¾ teaspoon sea salt

½ teaspoon freshly ground **black pepper**

½ teaspoon **cayenne** or chipotle **chile powder**

Preheat the oven to 425 degrees F. Line a baking sheet with parchment paper or a silicone baking mat.

Put all the ingredients in a large bowl and stir until the sweet potatoes are evenly coated. Transfer to the lined baking sheet and spread into a single layer. Bake for 20 minutes.

Remove from the oven. Stir, then spread out the sweet potatoes to form a single layer again. Bake for 15 to 20 minutes longer, or until crisp and lightly browned around the edges. Serve hot.

Raw Stone Fruit Crumble

Makes 4 servings

This no-bake fruit crumble is ideal for hot summer months. Using very ripe fruit is a must for this dessert.

½ cup **coconut water** or water

6 pitted soft dates

1 cup raw **walnuts** or other nuts

⅓ cup unsweetened shredded dried **coconut**

1 teaspoon ground **cinnamon**

¼ teaspoon freshly grated nutmeg

4 **nectarines** or **peaches**, or 3 cups sliced **apricots**, **plums**, or **pluots**

1 teaspoon vanilla extract

½ teaspoon ground **ginger** or **cardamom**

Put the coconut water and dates in a small bowl. Set aside for 10 minutes to rehydrate the dates.

To make the crumble mixture, put four of the dates and the walnuts, coconut, cinnamon, and nutmeg in a food processor. Pulse until the mixture resembles coarse bread crumbs. Transfer to a small bowl and set aside.

To make the sauce, dice one of nectarines and put it in the food processor. If using sliced fruit, use 1 cup for the sauce. Add the vanilla extract, ginger, and the remaining two dates (save the soaking liquid) and process into a slightly chunky purée. Scrape down the work bowl. Continue processing, adding some of the soaking liquid as needed, until the mixture is smooth and saucy.

To assemble the crumble, slice the remaining 3 nectarines and put them in a 9-inch baking pan. Pour the sauce over the top and stir to evenly coat the fruit. Sprinkle the crumble mixture evenly over the top. Serve immediately or well chilled.

About the Author

Beverly Lynn Bennett is a seasoned vegan chef, baker, and writer who is passionate about showing the world how easy, delicious, and healthy a plant-based diet can be. Beverly is the author of numerous books, including *Almond Flour, Spiralize!, Kale: The Nutritional Powerhouse, CHIA,* and *Vegan Bites.*

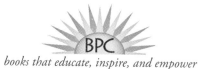

books that educate, inspire, and empower

All titles in the **Live Healthy Now** series are only **$5.95!**

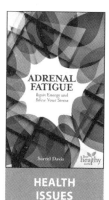
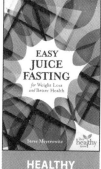
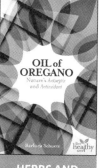
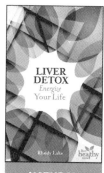

HEALTH ISSUES	HEALTHY FOODS	HERBS AND SUPPLEMENTS	NATURAL SOLUTIONS

Norman Walker's **COLON HEALTH**

SUGAR DETOX Defeat Cravings and Restore Your Health

THE ACID-ALKALINE DIET Balancing the Body Naturally

GLUTEN-FREE Success Strategies

A Holistic Approach to **ADHD**

Understanding **GOUT**

WHEAT BELLY Is Modern Wheat Causing Modern Ills?

KALE The Nutritional Powerhouse

Enhance Your Health with **FERMENTED FOODS**

GREEN SMOOTHIES The Easy Way to Get Your Greens

PALEO Smoothies

Refreshing Fruit and Vegetable **SMOOTHIES**

OLIVE LEAF EXTRACT The Mediterranean Healing Herb

AROMATHERAPY Essential Oils for Healing

The Pure Power of **MACA**

HERBAL ANTIVIRALS for Boosting Immunity

Ehret's **MUCUSLESS DIET**

The Healing Power of **TURMERIC**

Weight Loss and Good Health with **APPLE CIDER VINEGAR**

Healthy and Beautiful with **COCONUT OIL**

The Weekend **DETOX**

Improve Digestion with **FOOD COMBINING**

See our complete line of titles at **BookPubCo.com**
or order directly from: BPC • PO Box 99
Summertown, TN 38483 • 1-888-260-8458
Free shipping on all book orders